First Kiss

Reasonable Doubts Is A Standalone Contemporary
Romance Novel That Includes An Additional Bad Boy
Romance Storyline

*(The Mastery Of Kissing: Emulating The Techniques Of A
Hollywood Film Star)*

BogdanŻuromski

The intense torrent of rain was providing much-needed relief from the humidity of the steamy morning. The enormous raindrops pelted the automobile windshields, slowing traffic to a crawl. Some drivers felt it was too unsafe to continue driving, so they pulled over and waited for the storm to lighten up.

Emily wasn't deterred by the storm, though. She was returning to Sherwood High School to meet one-on-one with every kid. She would have the opportunity to get to know them better then. It was the final stage before she finalized her decision and sent Mary at work an email with it.

Since the school was closed for summer break, getting a spot near the door was simple. She reached into the passenger seat beside her, grabbed her bag, and secured it over her shoulder before retrieving her umbrella. She pushed the umbrella up and slid out of the car after opening the door.

Emily hurried to the front of the building, where a security guard was waiting to hold a door open, relieved that she hadn't been too wet.

"Oh my god. I sincerely appreciate you letting me in. As she shut the umbrella and entered, she stated, "I would have gotten soaked to the bone if I had to stop to ring the bell."

"Ms. Bawler, it's not a problem," the young lady remarked. "Mrs. Fidel informed me that you were on your way, and given the unfavorable weather today, I decided to come up and make sure you were okay."

Emily remarked, "Well, I thank you anyhow," as she removed her jacket. "Mrs. Fidel, is she in her office?"

Indeed. I should send you in straight away, she said. The guard nodded toward an open door on her left and stated, "The kids are there too."

"Excellent," exclaimed Emily as she moved in the direction the guard had indicated with a nod. "And once more, thank you."

The woman grinned and replied, "Not a problem," before settling behind the front desk.

Emily grinned at herself for being a few minutes early as she looked at the wall-mounted clock. Being late was something she detested. She would always feel unworthy or untrustworthy as a result.

She reached the open entrance and tapped on the glass door with her hand.

"Mrs. Fidel?"

Grinning, Mrs. Fidel looked up from her task. She stood and said, "Ms. Bawler, please come in."

Emily entered and was immediately struck by the abundance of ribbons, trophies, and achievement plaques in the showcase cabinet, which took up the entire right side of the space. Beautiful brass decorations adorned it, and brilliant lights shone on the prizes. It was Mrs. Fidel's pride and joy, of course.

Emily, who knew she wasn't late, added, "I hope I didn't keep you waiting too long."

"No, no, no. Even though I'm usually here early, you arrive on schedule. The children are waiting over there in the conference room. They had barely completed breakfast when I delivered it to them.

Mrs. Fidel approached Emily's desk and gave her two folders. These were bigger than the ones she gave her at the group home recital. Emily was excited to read all their files as soon as she realized she had them.

She gestured to a coat hook on the wall and added, "You can leave your jacket here." This shouldn't require much time at all. I know you will ask the kids a few questions before choosing. However, I must let you know that Khandace is not feeling well this morning before you enter. She's tough and won't tell me what's wrong with her. Tell me if you feel you can't handle her for whatever reason, and I'll take her away.

"I comprehend. Let me begin with Donald. Emily speculated that might provide her a little more time to calm down.

Thanking Emily for understanding, Mrs. Fidel smiled and touched her shoulder.

"It seems like a really good idea."

They went inside the well-lit room together. Sitting on one side of the table, Donald perused through a music book. When Emily went looking for Khandace, she discovered the young woman playing a game on her phone while concealed behind a pile of chairs.

"All right, boys. Donald, Ms. Bawler is here, and she will begin with you. Khandace, please accompany me.

Khandace scowled as she looked up. "Why are you starting with him instead of me?"

Mrs. Fidel started to say something, but Emily spoke first.

"Because in the alphabet D comes before K."

Emily only looked at her, offering no other explanation. Khandace got to her feet gradually and grabbed her book bag. She kept looking at her while moving in her direction. She turned her head away upon realizing Emily would not back down.

Mrs Fidel breathed a sigh of relief. She feared they would have a major falling out and that Ms. Bawler would never want to see her again. If all goes well, they might attract the interest of other universities, who might then begin to recruit some of their pupils for academic programs.

Emily turned to Donald after seeing Khandace and Mrs. Fidel exit the room. She placed her bag and the folders on the table and sat across from him. She took everything she required out of her purse, then settled back and grinned.

"Donald, are you ready to start?"

"Yes," he answered in a monotone.

Alright, alright.

Emily put down her pen and excused herself from Donald after twenty minutes.

That's all, Donald. You're free to leave. Please bring in Khandace as you are leaving.

Indeed.

His bland "yes" answer to her again made Emily giggle almost to tears. She observed him lift his fitting hat and give him a backhand slap on his head. Then he picked up an umbrella and walked to the entrance.

Khandace entered the office shortly after he left. She moved to take the seat that Donald had just cleared out. She threw her luggage beside her and slumped back into her chair, looking bored.

Emily grabbed her academic sheet as soon as she opened the folder. Precisely like she had imagined, she was gifted and had potential, according to her teachers, but her actions prevented her from realizing it. Fortunately, there was a simple way through that obstacle. Identify the core of the issue.

Emily closed the folder and grabbed her pen and a blank questionnaire form. She cast a glance at Khandace and thought of something.

She looked at the folder and said, "Is that folder about me?"

"Yes."

Her eyes were sharp as she gazed at the folder. "What's contained within?"

"Almost everything you have done since the first grade."

Her eyes met Khandace's.

"Is my private information contained therein?"

After glancing at the folder, Emily turned back to face her.

"A few."

She averted her gaze and shook her head.

Emily remained silent. She wants to hold off on her. She had had a rough morning, and Emily didn't want to put her through further stress.

She asked, her eyes fixed on the rain outside the window, "Don't you have some questions on that paper to ask me or something?"

Indeed, I do. But first, allow me to ask you a question.

Khandace avoided glancing at her.

Do you desire this? Because if you don't, you are free to leave, and we can end this immediately.Khandace, hurry up. Persuade me that you desire this.

With a sudden start, Khandace got up and pushed her chair aside. She attempted to grab her bag, but it was entangled in the chair's legs. She screamed in frustration after struggling with the bag for a short while and failing to get it loose.

When she opened the door, Emily talked to Mrs. Fidel without looking at her. "Mrs. Fidel, our interview is still ongoing. Please wait for me to call before you return. She tried to lessen the impact of her words as she said, "Thank you.

Khandace had just managed to free her suitcase when Mrs. Fidel slammed the door. Emily merely sat there, observing her as she went around the table.

Khandace, hurry up. Speak up!

Khandace was furious for a while. "Let me tell you something! "That garbage you have in that folder does not define who I am," she cried. Anger heaved in her chest.

"It doesn't,"

"No! Not by a long shot. These snobby ass teachers don't listen to you; they just act like they do. They misrepresent you and include untrue and misleading statements. Getting the check is all that matters to them.

"So what's the real story?" quietly inquired Emily.

"What?" That was not a question she was ready for.

Emily got up and came over to her. Now, there was hardly a space between them as they stood face to face.

"Please tell me the real story of Khandace Murphy."

Silently, Khandace stood there. Her muscles tensed with repressed rage.

With a tear streaming down her cheek, she exclaimed aggressively, "You want to know the truth?"

"Yes," Emily replied earnestly. "I desire the actual truth. Not the nonsense that's in that folder. Tell me about yourself.

"All right," she nodded. Alright. Okay, I need it.

"What is it that you need?"

There were more tears.

"It! The music! I require it. I simply do, and I'm not sure why. You know, it's helpful.

"It aids with what?"

Khandace put her head down and squeezed closed her eyes. Her tiny hands clenched around her bag's strap.

"All of it," she muttered. "All of it. It muffles the sound. It ends the suffering. It prevents me from seeing my life's despair and hopelessness. Emily looked up and saw a young person tortured by the life that poverty and a lack of healthy influences had put upon her.

Emily questioned, "Why did you choose music?"

Khandace tossed her purse onto a chair next to the entrance.

As she turned to go, she questioned, "Why did I choose music?" With a hollow laugh, she wiped her damp face. "Dude, I didn't select the music." It picked me out. "What do you mean?" Emily approached her again.

I was taken to the music room and detained for toppling the cafeteria garbage can. I wanted to smash the violin when I saw it sitting there. Nevertheless, I unintentionally strung the strings when I lifted it. I hesitated at that sound, you know. I had a strange feeling.

"I picked up the bow after noticing it sitting there. I can still picture people playing on TV and lifting it to my shoulder. She turned to face Emily. "I felt foolish at first. I had to check to make sure I was not being watched. I then got inside the game. Have fun.

Her laugh sounded forced, though. Void.

As you can see, I never studied music notation or took lessons. I used to skip music class because I thought it was boring. How, then, did I accomplish that? Even now, I'm still unsure how I achieved it. Why did I find it so easy to pick up music reading skills?

"You can, Khandace."

"No, Ms. Bawler, you don't understand." She took a step toward her. "I promised to be honest with you about myself. In actuality, it's everything—not just the violin.

Emily continued her explanation as she stood there looking perplexed.

"I don't know how, but I can play the guitar, saxophone, flute, and piano. She broke down in tears, saying, "I think I'm some sort of freak or something."

With a smile, Emily extended her arm to embrace her. Indeed!

She felt her settle into her arms after a few minutes of holding her. Then she drew her to a chair, grabbing her by the hand. Satisfied with the silence, they took a seat close to one another.

"Hear me out, Khandace. You're not strange. Emily took her hand and lifted her chin when she didn't answer. "Have you heard me?" You're not strange. But I am aware of who you are.

Khandace appeared anxious. "It seems like there's a problem with me?"

Emily shook her head, grinning. "No, you're simply unique. What you are has a name among them. Prodigy.

"What exactly is a prodigy?"

It's a person endowed with extraordinary traits or skills, particularly if they are young. For you, it is melody. You can play almost any instrument you pick up because of this. That explains why you find learning to read music so simple. And that's the reason you think you need it so badly. It now forms a part of your existence. You're not weird, Khandace. You are truly remarkable.

Khandace glanced at her hands as though she had never seen them before. Emily was shocked when she looked up.

She had never seen the girl grin before, and she was too cute for words.

Emily grinned back, "I hope that smile means you won't be kicking over chairs any more."

Khandace laughed. Yes, I apologize for that. I was quite unhappy and perplexed as I didn't know what was happening to me.

You'll discover how to transfer that vigor and feeling into your songs. It becomes less difficult.

"Yes, I suppose so."

"Oh, how disappointing. Examine the time. It's been nearly thirty-five minutes since we started talking. Emily replied as she stood up, "I didn't want to keep you so long.

It's okay, Khandace reassured. "At least the rain stopped."

Emily quickly glanced out the window, "Yes, that's true."

While Khandace gathered her book bag, Emily returned to the table and organized her belongings. At the door, they both met.

"Thank you so much for everything, Ms. Bawler. Most importantly, For listening to me and clarifying things for me. Although I know I won't receive the scholarship, I don't mind. Donald is deserving. Since he was a little child, he has played. In any case, many thanks.

"Thank you very much," Emily said as Khandace slid out the doorway.

As Emily left the room, Mrs. Fidel hurried in and nearly ran into her.

"Oh! I apologize. I was unaware that you were at the door," she remarked as she peered around. "Is everything okay?"

Indeed, everything is good. Emily moved by her to pick up her umbrella from the ground and her jacket off the rack. I'll get in touch with you shortly to discuss my choice. Since I know you might not be present, I'll drop over in person to give Principal Vox the scholarship documents.

Mrs. Fidel started to grin. "I'm overjoyed that everything happened as planned. Perhaps there will be more pupils for you to grade next year.

Emily grinned. "Perhaps." After that, she grabbed her purse and walked out of the office.

Emily walked out of the building, shaking her head at the bizarre weather in Virginia. The outdoors looked like it was about to get hurricane season this morning, but now that the sun was out, the birds were singing, and the humidity was attempting to damage her hair. Neither a jacket nor an umbrella was necessary anymore.

She descended the school's stairs and exclaimed, "Good Lord, this heat is awful."

"Emily, hello."

Emily whirled around in shock to discover Sherry at the bottom of the stairs.

How in the hell? "Sherry? Why are you in this place?

Sherry had waited to see Emily again for days in her car, where she could still see the entrance to the school after losing Emily in traffic. She hurried over to welcome her as soon as she noticed her stride emerge from the building.

She eased up one step at a time and added, "Oh, I was in the neighborhood."

"The local area?" Uneasy, Emily shifted to her right. "Are you aware of anyone who attends this school?" she questioned skeptically.

Sherry raised Emily's question as if it had never occurred to her. "Given your presence, may I inquire whether you would be interested in joining me for lunch? Something Italian, perhaps? She smiled and remarked, "I know you enjoy Italian cuisine.

How in the world is she aware of that? I'm sorry, but no. I have to be somewhere right now. She started to down the stairs, keeping a safe distance from her.

Sherry's joy vanished when she heard Emily turn down her offer once more. "You enjoy playing games with me, don't you?" she questioned as she observed Emily turning to go.

Emily paused and pivoted, agitated. "Pardon me? Engaging in gaming. What the devil kind of game am I playing with you? We're not in a relationship. I have no desire to date you. Sherry, you should avoid me at all costs. What you anticipate transpiring between us is not going to occur. Don't bother talking to me the next time you see me. Act as though you don't even know who I am.

Emily turned and went in the direction of her car after that. Sherry was nowhere to be seen when she glanced back over her shoulder. She went to her car and got behind the wheel, upset that she had to correct her. She was so enraged that Sherry dared to suggest that they were acting like they were dating. She was so angry that she neglected to glance in the rearview mirror, where she would have noticed Sherry trailing behind her.

The afterglow of our first encounter

We were suffering from the aftereffects of our newfound intimacy as we returned to our separate houses, and it felt wonderful. Our conversations were revitalized and became more intimate, sensual, and horny. Even though I was having a fantastic time, I wondered if everything would be this simple. Was it that simple to receive a kiss or have a female accept you? There were moments when nothing made sense. I wasted much of my graduation year pursuing girls to win them over. It was strange; I still remember the people who rejected me and the jokes I made about myself. How every time someone of the other sex rejected me, my buddies would make fun of me. However, I'm not sure why. Whether it was my sex hormones or my dying spirit, I would brush away those hurtful sentiments of rejection and start over. And here I was, barely attempting,

A pretty attractive and seductive girl in her own right says, "Wow, I'm romantic."

It was simultaneously lovely and strange.

But putting aside all of the butterflies in my stomach and the positive emotions rushing through me like cola bottle foam. I had a gut feeling that something wasn't right. I sensed somewhere that it was not meant to be. I understood that my feelings for this girl were not sincere, but a thief was hiding in my thoughts since an affair had finally occurred. Even if it meant that the female got wounded in the process, I considered just going with the flow. Even so, I prayed to the gods above, hoping She wouldn't become serious.

We resumed our conversation, and I soon realized she was in complete awe of me and giving me love beyond measure. I loved it more than anything because she had turned into such a romantic, but that's also when my inner anxiety took over, and I started to become cautious. I suppose a dating rule—possibly a worldwide one—states that once one party in a relationship shows too much affection, the other partner becomes wary or begins to play it safe.

It's a phenomenon that couples all over the world have noticed. Every time you lose yourself in them, they treat you casually, with a dash of sweetness and salt. In my situation, she pursued attention while I received it all. I was having so much fun, even though I was afraid, but I would push it away.

I returned to college when the Dussehra holidays came to a close. Back to my hectic days, but this time, I felt like I had changed. I felt happier, more at ease, and appeared to be lost. I was also fantasizing a little more. The observers saw a pleasing inconsistency in me. It felt like I was living my best life because I was comfortable with myself. The reality is that even though I might have been exaggerating things because it was all new to me, her sexually suggestive humor would make me giggle uncontrollably late at night. I would never stop thinking about her during the day.

Even though we had hectic daily schedules, I was preparing for our next event, and she was preparing for a competitive exam. Even so, we would make time to indulge each other's sex cravings.

It was clear from our first date that we were eager to be together again, yet managing our hormones was not always simple due to our busy schedules. I recall seeing this Ramleela poster featuring DeepikaPadukone and Ranveer Singh while we were returning from viewing Lunchbox. She declared that we would see this and was excited to watch it. Our hormones were exploding during the period when Ramleela was supposed to happen. We needed to meet, but the questions of how and when to do so needed to be answered.

As usual, I had a part to play in our group's musical drama that we would present at the Diwali Inter College celebration, which was quickly approaching. As a result, I got busy with our rehearsals. She became preoccupied with her daily lectures and lessons, and it was during this hectic timetable that we eventually managed to find a brief moment to speak. My rehearsals ended at 2:30 on Saturdays, while her lessons ended at two. Ahoy, That implied that we had nearly two hours to work with. By 5:30, her mother would return home, meet me, and head home. Now that we had located the window, it was time to choose a location for our conversation.

After giving it some thought, she chose the location herself, and it was a park close to her campus. A public park, though a little remote. My eyes widened as I realized that public parks are often deserted at lunchtime. And I was anticipating a lot of very personal behavior.

I was energized from the start of that personal day, living in a different reality where I was content and experiencing the jitters and highs of emotion.

That coziness and good-natured feeling.

My pals quickly sensed that something was off, and the girls in my gang also quickly realized I was seeing someone. Girls are intelligent beings who can detect emotions and date well; I'm not sure why we call them stupid. And I heard them ask, "What's the deal? Someone is lost here today." All I needed to do to make myself blush was Anoop and those playful moments. Oh my, It was so satisfying. Though my gangmates began to feel the same way, they had no idea what was happening until I began showing them a little more bromance with my embraces. Love does that to you, doesn't it? It truly makes you adore everything around you— everything that comes your way—and I experienced the same thing.

Even though I still had the nagging feeling that something wasn't right, I was losing the plot as I was embraced in intimacy.

Next, we shared a kiss.

As I practiced thinking of her, time passed quickly, and I noticed the time on my phone was two o'clock. I have to get out, I decided. I told my group, while they were all laying their asses on the ground that we had to depart a little early today because I had some work to do. My friends started teasing me, saying, "Oh, you're going on a date?" What the heck, I thought; how did they find out? I suppose I did give away all the clues with my facial expressions. I had to get out as quickly as possible, so who cares? The girls smiled mischievously at me as I said goodbye to them, and my brothers still had no idea what was happening.

Since I was late the last time and didn't want to make the same mistake again, I rode my bike as fast as possible. I also needed to freshen myself since, after all those practices and the sweat that seeped through my armpits, I'm sure my scent wasn't attractive enough for someone to want to embrace me. And I yearned to feel her amazing scent, to feel her embrace me and get close to me. I had to shower quickly to accomplish all that, so I did that as soon as I got home. After changing into a new T-shirt and applying deo to my underarms, I hurried to the park, where she awaited me. It was 2.45, and I knew I would be late again. I simply hoped she would forgive me. Screw it.

She sat on her active, listening to tunes and killing time as I arrived at the intended intimate spot. I silently parked my bike behind her and approached her to give her a cheerful shock, sliding gently toward her like a serpent pursuing its victim. To my amazement, though, she remarked, "I knew it the moment you had arrived," and she remained unfazed. Try this trick again another time; it's quite ancient. I said, "Oh no, I just missed it by a tiny bit." Based on my reactions, the girls in my group seemed to know that I would be going on a date. Was I so brutally honest when I arrived? These days, what has happened to honesty? I shook my thoughts aside, wondering if she would ever discover that I was not really into her, even if I gave out so many clues. She took me into the park as we arrived. While we were looking for a cozy, appropriate spot to relax, she said, "How come you are always late, Mr. Busy?" I just apologized and told her I would be on time the next time because I had nothing more to say, and I knew it wouldn't be worth it. You see, there's always another time. I gave her a wink when I said this.

She lightly punched me in the elbow.

I laughed out loud.

As I assessed her, she looked stunning in her blue trousers and scarlet top. She swung her buttocks as she walked, and it felt fantastic to look there. Just as I was getting pleasure from her swaying hips, she abruptly stopped, took my hand, and guided me over to a bench. After some slight hustling, she had found a bench at last. Together, we strolled to our preferred bench. We sat there, hands clasped, staring at one another. The bench was well situated, directly under a large tree. In addition, it appeared to be the ideal romantic environment because it was shaded, and the leaves were dropping regularly. I've never felt the afternoon so lovely.

Her long hair billowed over her face, sultry eyes and slightly pink lips drew my attention. She was stunning and alluring. I took hold of her waist, drew her in, and kissed her on both cheeks. She applied a firm, stinging pinch on my arms. My mouth ached a little bit at that point. She looked at me, turning her eyes. I tell you, that look was pure evil. It confused me more than it scared me. She continued with that same wicked stare,

"You're quite desperate, mister Haan."
Baby, keep your hands to yourself. At that warning, I laughed and responded, Alright.

Then, she started talking to me, telling me about her college days and hoping she could learn to dance. I silently took her hands and started to play with her fingers while giving her hands intermittent kisses while she continued to murmur. She answered a call from a buddy in the middle of everything, but she was preoccupied. As she spoke with a buddy about filling out an exam form, I had a chance to look closely at her. As I drew closer, I could see her gorgeous cleavage and her velvety bra beneath her red top. I was seeing them up close for the first time, and they were incredible. Her fragrance was so enticing that I wanted to rub my face all over her. I was searching for a means to accomplish that when I saw her college ID card hanging around her neck and had an epiphany. I picked it up and slowly began stroking her body below her neck in strange ways. Gently, move circularly. She put up a fight until she lost control, at which point she reached for my right thigh and disconnected the call.

Her breathing had become labored.

Her body odor was very intoxicating, as were her breaths.

I embraced her, brushed her hair aside, and kissed her lips. We met eye contact, and as I drew forward, she moved in closer, kissed me, and closed her eyes.

This occurred independently, seemingly in a river-like flow across the valleys. Oh, I tell you, I lost control after those private activities. She grabbed my hair and slid her hands across my head. Our lips slowly touched each other as it started. It continued endlessly. I was completely lost on another planet. We were examining one other's private taste buds with our tongues. Both the wildness and beauty of that moment were present. I'm not sure how much time it lasted. However, we were so out of breath that we tore our lips apart. She covered her face and shouted, "What did we just do?" blushing with happy embarrassment as I glanced at her. I inquired, "How was it?" "SHUT UP," she uttered. In that fleeting moment, she looked so adorable that I embraced her. It was quiet. All I wanted was time to stand still and that particular moment to remain unchanged. My first KISS was that one. I took her hands as she laid her head on my shoulder. Even the environment around us seemed arousing, in my opinion. She slid her hands over my body and unbuttoned my shirt—I'm not sure what triggered her. She started stroking my chest. She seemed to be playing a joke on me, saying, "So now you understand how it feels when you do this to me," as the pleasure began to shoot through my spine, giving me intense erotic vibrations. She descended. She replied, "Wow, Baby, my kiss made you pregnant, haa," as she caressed my stomach. She bowed and pressed her ears to my belly, saying, "Let me hear our baby's heartbeats." Our baby is inside you. "What nonsense, you are crazy..ha ha hahahahaha," I exclaimed. She laughed out loud, as well as me. Together, we let out a big laugh.

We had used up all our time as we sat together for a while longer. Now that it was five o'clock, it was time for her to go. She got up to go, but I was unable to follow her. She gave me an odd look. How the fuck do you look? I remarked, "The erection is still there, and I cannot stand up. There is this bump showing up on my jeans," as I looked at her hopelessly. What the heck, she thought, and she sat by my side, tending to me tenderly. Thank you, but I said that won't be of any use. Yeah, I said, and she was like, what? Simply avoid sitting so close, and everything will become more relaxed. She laughed the hardest she had ever laughed at that.

When I got home, I realized I had completely lost the plot. Now, I was dependent on her.

I was fascinated with her at this point, having been addicted to the sensual pleasure she was providing.

I had been overly into her for a while, but suddenly, I was aloof. I use her as a stress reliever now. I would continue talking to her even after balancing homework and practicing with my friends for our next musical theater. And she would make me giggle all day long. I wanted to text through my schedule, so it felt quite natural. I was having a great time doing everything and strolling around content. I felt fantastic doing even the most ordinary activities.

The March
The Car of Henry - October 2017
After dragging me out of the sanctuary, Henry sat me down on the sidewalk outside of our former Sunday school classroom and held me on his lap until I was no longer crying.
He threw me into his car and drove off, leaving me to wretch and
The fallout from our initial meeting

We were back at our separate houses, suffering from the aftereffects of our newfound intimacy, and it felt amazing.

We had more intimate, sensual, and lustful chats as a result of our renewed energy. Though loving it, I privately questioned whether it would all be this easy. Was it that easy to be kissed and accepted by a woman? There were times when logic failed to occur. I chased females and tried to win them over for part of my graduation year. It was weird; I could still recall my jokes about myself and the people who rejected me. How my friends would make fun of me every time I got turned down by someone of the opposite sex. I'm not sure why, though. Whether it was my dying soul or my sex hormones, I would push those bitter feelings of rejection aside and start afresh. And here I was, barely even trying to

A girl on the verge of becoming a woman declares, "Wow, I'm romantic."

It was odd and beautiful at the same time.

Nevertheless, I forced myself to ignore the happy feelings and butterflies in my stomach that were racing through me like cola bottle foam. I sensed that something wasn't quite right. Somewhere inside me, I knew it was not meant to be. Since an affair had finally happened, I realized my affection for this girl was not genuine, but a thief was lurking in my mind. I thought about going with the flow, even if it meant the woman got hurt in the process. Nevertheless, I prayed to the higher gods, hoping she wouldn't get serious.

When we started talking again, I quickly realized she was utterly enthralled with me and showed me unfathomable affection. She had become such a romantic, and I loved it more than anything, but that's also when my inner nervousness took over, and I began to become cautious. It's probably a universal dating law that when one person in a relationship expresses too much affection, the other partner gets cautious or starts to play it safe.

Couples from all around the world have observed this occurrence. Every time you lose yourself in them, they handle you carelessly, with a hint of sweetness and salt. In my case, I was getting all the attention, and she was the one seeking it.

Despite my fear, I was having a great time but would ignore it.

When the Dussehra holidays ended, I went back to college. I returned to my busy days but felt like I had evolved. I looked lost, felt more content, and relaxed. And I was daydreaming a bit more. I had a nice irregularity that the onlookers noticed. I was so at ease with who I was that I felt like I was living my best life. The truth is that her sexually suggestive humor would make me laugh uncontrollably late at night, and I would never stop thinking about her during the day, even though I might have been exaggerating things because it was all new to me.

We both had busy daily schedules, but in between, I was preparing for our next event, and she was preparing for a competitive exam. We would still schedule a time to satiate our sexual desires together.

We were excited to get together again after our first date, but because of our hectic schedules, controlling our hormones wasn't always easy. I distinctly remember seeing this poster for Ramleela, which starred Ranveer Singh and DeepikaPadukone, on the way back from lunch. She said, eager to see it, "We're definitely going to see this." When Ramleela was meant to happen, our hormones were erupting. We had to get together but also figure out when and how to accomplish it.

As usual, I was involved in our group's musical theater, which we would perform at the Diwali Inter College festival, which was drawing near. I consequently became preoccupied with our rehearsals. She got caught up in her regular lectures and classes, and in the midst of this busy schedule, we finally found a few minutes to talk. Her lessons concluded at two, but my Saturday rehearsals ended at 2:30. That meant we would have over two hours to work with. Her mother would be home by 5:30, greet me, and then go back. Now that we knew where the window was, it was time to decide where our talk would take place. After careful consideration, she picked the spot, a park near her university. It's a little isolated but a public park. When I noticed public parks were frequently empty around lunch, my eyes widened. And I was expecting a great deal of highly intimate activity.

From the beginning of that private day, I felt invigorated and content, being in a completely other world and going through emotional highs and lows.

That warmth and kind feeling.

The girls in my gang also quickly discovered I was seeing someone, and my friends instantly sensed something was wrong. I'm not sure why we label girls as stupid; they're clever individuals who can sense emotions and make good dates. I then heard someone inquire, "What's the matter? There's a lost person here today." All I had to do was look at Anoop and those carefree times and blush. Oh my, It was fulfilling. My gangmates started to feel the same way, but they didn't realize it until I started giving them a little more bromance through my embraces. That's what love does to you, isn't it? It does make you love everything around you and everything that comes your way. This is exactly what happened to me.

I was losing the plot as I felt the intimacy of being caressed, even though I still had that nagging feeling that something wasn't right.

We then exchanged kisses.

Time flew by while I practiced thinking of her, and I saw that my phone was showing the hour as two o'clock. I made up my mind to leave. While everyone was kicking themselves on the ground, I informed my group that we had to leave early today because I needed to finish some work. I was being teased by my pals, who would say things like, "Oh, you're going on a date?" How the hell did they find out, I wondered. With my facial expressions, I guess I did reveal every hint. Who cares? I had to get out as fast as I could. When I bid farewell to the females, they gave me a naughty look, and my brothers were still completely clueless about what was happening.

I rode my bike quickly because I didn't want to repeat my previous late error. I also needed to shower because I'm sure my smell wasn't appealing enough for someone to want to hug me after all those practices and the sweat that leaked through my armpits. And I yearned to be near her, to feel her lovely aroma, and to feel her embrace me. To do that, I had to take a quick shower, which I did as soon as I arrived home. I raced to the park where she awaited me, putting video on my underarms and changing into a fresh T-shirt. It was 2.45 by now, and I knew I would be late again. All I could do was hope she would pardon me. Forget about it.

When I got to the designated intimacy area, she sat quietly, enjoying music and passing the time. I parked my bike secretly behind her and glided softly toward her, like a snake chasing its prey, to give her a happy shock. She said, "I knew it the moment you had arrived," to my surprise, and she didn't seem to be phased. This is an old trick, so give it another go. "Oh no, I just missed it by a tiny bit," was my reaction. My reactions gave the impression that the girls in my group knew I would be going on a date. Was I so ruthlessly honest when I first got here? What happened to honesty these days? Even though I was giving her a lot of hints, I wondered whether she would ever figure out that I was not really into her. I brushed my thoughts aside. When we got to the park, she led me inside. She said, "How come you are always late, Mr. Busy?" as we searched for a comfortable, suitable place to unwind. I had nothing more to say and realized it wouldn't be worth it, so I just apologized and promised her I would be on time the next time. There's always another time, you see. When I stated this, I winked at her.

She gave me a gentle elbow punch.

I let out a loud laugh.

I thought she looked amazing in her red top and blue pants as I examined her. As she moved, she swayed her buttocks, and it felt great to stare there. I was enjoying the sensation of her swinging hips when she stopped quickly, held my hand, and led me to a bench. Finally, after a little hustle, she had located a bench. We walked to our favorite bench together. With our hands clenched, we sat there gazing at each other. The bench was ideally positioned beneath a big tree. It was also shaded, and with the leaves falling often, it seemed like the perfect setting for a passionate affair. The afternoon has never felt so beautiful to me.

I was drawn in by her sensual eyes, slightly pink lips, and long hair that flowed over her face. She was attractive and seductive. I grabbed her waist, pulled her in, and kissed her on the cheek. She pinched my arms hard, making them sting. That's when my mouth started to hurt a little. She turned her head to gaze at me. That gaze was pure wickedness, I assure you. I was more perplexed by it than afraid. "Mister Haan, you're quite desperate," she said, fixing him with that same icy gaze. Baby, please don't touch me. I laughed at that warning and said, "Okay."

She then spoke with me about her first day of college and her desire to pick up dancing. She kept murmuring, so I took her hands and silently began to play with her fingers, kissing her hands now and again. Amidst all this, she took a call from a friend, but she was distracted. She was talking to a friend about filling out an exam form when I got a chance to glance her over. Her red top was covered in a silky bra and stunning cleavage, which I could see as I got closer. They were amazing, and I was seeing them up close for the first time. Her smell drew me in, making me want to rub my face all over her. I was looking for a way to do that and had a lightbulb moment when I noticed her college ID card hanging around her neck. I took it up and slowly started giving her odd body caressing motions below her neck. Move in a gentle, gentle circular motion. She fought till she became uncontrollable, then she grabbed my right thigh and ended the call.

She was having trouble breathing.

Her breath and body odor were intoxicating.

I hugged her, pushed her hair to the side, and kissed her. We made eye contact, and she went in closer, kissed me, and closed her eyes as I drew forward. Everything happened as if it were flowing across the valleys like a river. Oh, I tell you, after those private exchanges, I lost control. She moved her hands across my head, grabbing my hair. It began with our lips slowly brushing against one another. It went on forever. I felt like I was in another world. We were using our tongues to probe each other's intimate taste buds. There was the beauty and the savagery of that moment. I had no idea how long that lasted. But we were so breathless that we were tearing our lips off. I gazed at her, and she covered her face, shouting, "What did we just do?" blushing with ecstatic humiliation. My question was, "How was it?" "Shut up," was all she said. She looked so cute in that brief period that I embraced her tightly. Everything was silent. I just wanted time to stop and one specific instant to stay unaltered. It was the first KISS I ever had. She rested her head on my shoulder, and I took her hands. I found the surroundings to be stimulating as well. I can't quite figure out what made her move to unbutton my shirt and slide her hands over my body. She began to caress my chest. "So now you understand how it feels when you do this to me," she said, perhaps pulling a practical joke on me as strong sensual vibrations started to shoot through my spine. She went downstairs. "Wow, Baby, my kiss made you pregnant, haa," she said, patting my belly. She put her hands on my belly, bent down, and said, "Let me hear our baby's heartbeats." Inside, you are our kid. "What nonsense, you are crazy..ha ha hahahahaha," I yelled. Both she and I let out a huge laugh. We both gave a hearty laugh.

We sat there together for a little longer until we had used up all our time. It was five o'clock now, and she should be heading out. She stood up to leave, but I could not catch up with her. She looked at me strangely. How do you look, dude?

"The erection is still there, and I can't get up," I said. There's this lump on my jeans," I said, staring hopelessly at her. What the heck, she thought, and she caressed me softly while sitting by my side. I said, "Thank you, but that won't help." Indeed, I replied, and she said, "What?" Just don't sit so close together, and things will settle down. That made her laugh harder than she had ever laughed.

I realized I had completely lost the narrative when I arrived home. I was completely reliant on her now.

At this time, I was addicted to the sensual pleasure she was giving me, and I was fascinated with her.

For a while, I had been tremendously attracted to her, but all of a sudden, it was me who was distant. I now utilize her as a way to decompress. Even after juggling my coursework and getting ready for our upcoming musical theater production with my friends, I would still be in contact with her. She also could make me laugh nonstop. It was natural to want to text through my schedule. I was wandering around happily, enjoying every moment of it all. I felt amazing performing even the most mundane tasks.

Feel sorry for yourself. Upon his return, accompanied by my mother, I realized that I had been blind to his behind-the-scenes scheming.

Knowing that Mom and Aggie would be with Danny's mother, I had walked to the church that morning to get a mile and some peace of mind. I was not prepared to meet her. Not quite yet. Perhaps never. However, Henry was waiting for me when I got to the church. He leaned against the structure and looked exactly like the child I had grown up with, save for a few more inches across his shoulders and chest.

And Henry had led me to a position in the back, away from as many prying eyes as possible (though I'd made that a pointless endeavor). His cool strength kept me from falling apart until even he was insufficient to confront my unbearable grief.

My mother turned to Henry as she bent over the front seat and kissed my cheek. "I'm grateful, sweetie. You wanted to be here for Jeremiah, I know that. It's a really difficult day for everyone.

My mother insisted that I keep it even though I had returned it more times than I could remember.

I was still spinning when my mother brought up the thing that disturbed me earlier. I swiveled in my chair to face her.

Was Lucy present? Henry was staring at the road when I returned to look at him. I turned back to the sole adult in the car who was still working, and all he could offer me was another clenching of the jaw. "Mum?"

"She didn't want to make Miriam sick on top of everything because she wasn't feeling well." At Henry's snort, she trailed off, and I whirled in shock. I prodded him since he was straining to maintain his cool cop façade. Hard.

Nothing in the world could prevent Lucy Keller from being by Mrs. Anderson's side today, short of a double amputation. Henry?

Jeremiah, quiet down. Henry is not involved in this at all! My mother's unwavering support of Henry wasn't all that absurd—after all, he was just another son to her—but when she insisted that Henry wasn't to blame in any way, it appeared there was some disagreement.

"She believes you're to blame for this?" Grabbing Henry's bicep, I attempted to persuade him to look at me. I felt thankful that we were now part of a convoy speeding through suburban streets at twenty miles per hour. With ease, he dismissed me, and once more, my mother responded on his behalf.

"Honey, nobody is to blame for it. Not even that of Danny. Undoubtedly not Henry's. He has helped the youngster more than a hundred saints could have, Lord knows.

She stepped forward, reaching out to give him a light grip on the shoulder. "Love, nobody believes this is your fault. Danny was tense and uneasy all the time. The only occasion I saw him calm down was when the three of you were together, even though he managed to hide it well under his charm regarding Lucy. She felt wounded because she was at the wrong place and time. It takes place. Now, when Miriam looks at her and at me and sees us with two grown, healthy, and, God forbid, alive sons, it breaks her heart. She needs time, but she will get over it. Her boy needs to be buried. Thus, it's fortunate that Agatha is with her.

Henry gave a firm nod, his eyes remaining focused on the automobile ahead of us, but his big, tan hand reached over my mother's light pink fingers hanging over his shoulder.

The words of adoration she had lavished onto Henry like a salve, as though it were the most natural thing in the world, amazed me.

Part One of The Cemetery, October 2017
Headstones were partially buried in drifts of crimson and gold in the frigid

graveyard. The groundskeepers appeared to be a practical group of people who would sooner wait to rake away what was left of autumn than keep watch.

Danny's burial place was framed by an upbeat carpet of synthetic grass lovingly cleared of leaves. There was an inconsiderate rush to complete the interment—especially after my performance—because of circumstances that even I didn't want to consider. There had been no viewing following the funeral.

There I was, my mother by my side and Aggie, who had given up on Mrs. Anderson to be with me. Based on my actions at the church, I wasn't sure if that meant the women's relationship had drastically changed or if it just meant that I was now seen as the more wounded one.

Henry stood to protect my flank, a foot behind me. His scarf curled around my throat as tight as my nerves, another one of his mothering gestures, and even though I was dressed up against the chill, I imagined I could feel his breath on the back of my neck. I squeezed back another tear and smelled the perfume in the felted material. Like the last time, I yearned for this day to end so I could dash to the airport and never look back.

The Last Days of Us

August 2003, Normal, Indiana

Driving on campus in Normal with my hatchback packed to the rafters, I had been excited. They had spent the previous day setting things up at the dorm. They called every several hours with updates, so I knew where to go. One day, I went AWOL and left everything in the car to tear across the grass.

Subsequently, I would scrutinize the situation and attempt to reconcile it with my response to comprehend the origin of my suffering. However, at that moment, I was acting entirely instinctively. Turning the corner, I noticed Danny around Henry and the two kissing intensely. My only choice was to take flight. I then took off running.

I'd never been able to keep anything from Henry, so I called Danny from the road and lied my ass off while leaning against a gas pump near Minneapolis.

I informed him that the University of Washington's writing department had always been my dream, that I had been waitlisted there, and that my admission had just arrived. I had to board a plane immediately to make orientation if I wanted the spot. His Henry would keep him from missing me. I'd return during the summer. Similar to earlier eras.

Though Danny didn't say anything, it sounded fake to me. Just in time, I hung up when I heard Henry in the background begging to talk on the phone. He was harder to trick than I was, so I didn't answer his calls until I got to Washington. I was worried that I would return if I heard Henry's voice pleading with me to.

My decision was solidified when I saw the blue waters of Puget Sound after traversing the Rockies. I stayed in Seattle for the following four years, nursing my wounds. Strangely enough, all those lies came true despite my promises to the contrary. Following my graduation, I withdrew.

The excuses came easily because none of us had the money to take a plane for a visit. Even at the cost of my sister and mother, the thought of Danny and Henry being happy together was still too unbearable. It was amusing that Danny was still using me as a pawn in his scheme of things after all these years.

Just in time, I caught his arm and pulled him toward me, keeping him upright. Only now, as his breath burnt my face and his free hand settled on my waist, drawing me closer to him, did I realize just how close we were.

I tremble and become still, unsure how to react to this impulse. My own treacherous heart thumping hard in my chest echoes in my ears.

I breathe often, simultaneously taking in air and his perfume's spicy aroma. Intriguingly, I sense a shielding sense of tranquility surrounding me. I'm enjoying this embrace and not at all disappointed by what's taking place.

His racing heartbeat is visible through the pulsating vein in his neck, and his rapid breathing spreads happy shivers across my skin. I could feel his icy fingers grazing my waist through my jacket as if it were not there. That or my over-emotion was causing me to have tactile hallucinations.

- Regards," Dan smiled and pulled away from his impulsive hug. Should we leave?

I take off my helmet from the bike and nod.

All the way home, I couldn't stop thinking. It's as though I don't know what's going on and I don't belong. I'm acting with civility and common sense in ways that I never would have in the past. I've crossed every limit and personal guideline imaginable in such a short period! It's astounding!

I kissed a stranger. Even if it was unintentional and his idea, I still can't help but feel that this kiss keeps me up at night. I went to a race and followed some weird omens. I became a mascot, a source of good fortune, and I committed to attend two more races just for laughs. I jumped on a stranger's bike and went to a remote club together.

Dear NeraNera, what's wrong with you?

- Here we are," Dan approaches the driveway behind his car. Alright, so I'll see you in three days? I'm hoping you are still aware of two other races.

As I get off the bike, I say, "All right, I'll be there.

Immediately feeling empty and cold, I removed my jacket and helmet and gave them to the stranger.

"Keep it, you'll get it back after the next race," he said with a wink before driving off and rolling down his helmet's window.

I felt like I was wolfing it down when I looked at Dan because I felt so alone and depressed. I return home with reluctance and enter the kitchen. Since lunchtime today, I have not even had a bite to put in my mouth, and I refuse to even look at the food. I want to go to sleep, or more accurately, I want to curl up in a cozy bed, hide under a blanket, and close myself off from the outside world.

And so I do; I enter the bedroom, collapse into the bed, and mentally relive the previous day's events.

I buried my nose in my pillow and smiled obligingly, recalling the journey and the black-eyed guy's embrace. Why, God, did he enter my life? To ruin my life, to prevent me from having a peaceful existence?

Thirteen

Awaiting the new race, I waited. I counted the days until the race like a gullible idiot, and the three days seemed to go on forever. But here I was, watching Drago draw ahead and squeezing my fists uncomfortably in the stands. I'm unsure if it's entirely my fault, but the guy was beginning to pull ahead of his rivals.

Could it be that the initial triumph was a coincidental event and that Dan clung to me like a rock, and it functioned like, perhaps, a placebo?

But the outcome stays the same: Dan prevails, moving one victory closer to qualifying.

"Drago, you never cease to amaze us!" the race leader exclaims. Once more, what's the secret, or will you reveal it to us?

The guy looks at me for a moment and smiles as the stands quiet down. I try not to smile back, but that smile makes everything in my chest turn to pressure.

"It's the same secret that everyone else has," Dan replies. "I got lucky." - You didn't have much luck prior, did you? - You finally found the one. The cyclist receives a shoulder pat from the announcer.

- I was only searching in the incorrect location," Dan smiled.

- Would you please present her to us?

"No," the guy shook his head, "a girl that extraordinary ought to be shielded from prying eyes and kept safe.

I want to cover my burning ears with my hair, but I blush with embarrassment. Even though I know that this is all just a show and that much of what is said is probably true, these words nonetheless make me feel good.

As we exit the track, my companion asks, "Are you all right?" and I begin searching for Dan.

However, he is not present. Why did I assume he would wait for me and take me somewhere again this time? It wasn't as though a contract existed.

I smiled and answered, "Yeah, I'm fine," but my heart raced. -Are you heading home right now? Is that the last choice made?

Yes, indeed! My friend teases me, "I'm going to the party with everyone else, and you stay at home to wither away!" before bidding me farewell with a hug and walking toward some guy's car.

When is she going to have time to meet someone?

I turned toward the bus station after quickly glancing at the leaving automobile. I believe I'll heed her counsel and long to be at home.

I hear Dan's voice behind me. -Where are you going?

The guy walks alongside me after swiftly catching up to me. When I see him, I get a ton of butterflies in my stomach, which may be frightening.

"Where's your bike?" I ask, gazing at the guy's face with a voice shaking with excitement.

He allowed me to retain his leather jacket, so he's wearing his typical sweatshirt today. His image had changed from that of a rebellious rocker to that of an attractive, gregarious man.

- Within the carport. "Today, I had somewhat different plans," he smirked.

What kind of arrangements? - I came across as a little too eager.

Adjusting the hood of his hoodie and taking his phone out of his pocket, the man says, "Spend the evening with my luck and thank it for helping me qualify."

You were sent to me by Chance, which is fantastic.

Possibility... Still, there's one thing he's right about. We would never have met without the letter accident and his revelation that he was a race car driver.

Alright, let's move." After I told Dan the letter tale, he led me to the same cafe where I was blushing. You're not into loud company, so let's start with some food.

Sort of Like a First Date, Alma

When I arrived at the pool, he was not there. Had he already departed? Perhaps he wasn't supposed to leave so late.

I found a nice place to stand far from the ugly old lamppost and dipped my feet into the warm pool. I could feel sweat from my armpit because it was so hot. Did I overlook applying deodorant? I scented my armpits after looking around. Oh my, I noticed him getting closer.

"Hi, Monkey. I said, "Nice hair." He felt it a little awkwardly.

"Hey," he said as he walked over and sat too close.

Under a glimmer of moonlight, he gave me a piercing look as though he was itching to bite me. My tummy was churning with butterflies once more.

"You went out, and your aunt gave you a hard time?" I asked to be helped to stabilize myself.

"Not really, no," he responded.

He gave me a long glance before averting his gaze. I swallowed and tucked my hair behind my ear while considering my next words. Aside from the humming of hundreds of air units running nonstop, everything was quiet. Nobody was visible; they were all presumably sheltering from the heat.

I said, "Do you like school?"

"Not too much," he remarked. He questioned, "I bet you have a 4.0 GPA."

"Point four, five," I uttered.

"How on earth is that possible?" "It's like getting 100 and ten percent on a test with one hundred questions," he remarked.

I responded, "Well, it's not the same; you get extra credit, which improves your

GPA. Your GPA is greater if you already have a four.

"I'm not too fond of school. It's cheesy and dull. I always get rid of it," he remarked.

"You ditch? What do you mean? Do you not wish to attend college? I sound so judgmental, boy.

Yes, I will enroll in college, but I won't merely show up to class every day in an attempt to give the teacher enough students to keep his job. I don't care about the teacher's lesson because he doesn't care about me," he remarked.

For me, that was a deal breaker. I had no desire to spend time with a dummy.

"Skipping classes will how will you get into college?" I pushed, growing irritated.

"It's not that hard to get into college," he declared.

"What? Not only does a strong SAT score not ensure admission, but solid grades are also necessary. Perhaps this man is just another dumb boy.

"I'm going to enroll in community college first, then transfer." "Community college admits everyone," he continued.

I asked, "Don't you think that's kind of mediocre?" "Just stopping by?"

I was infuriated when he remarked, "Just because you find meaning in school doesn't mean it's important." "This is only high school." This con is a holdover from the industrial era. A method of turning farmers into manufacturing laborers. He sprayed some water on me. Some got into my eye.

Hey, please don't, I said.

"Go past who you are." He splashed more, yet again. He soaked my T-shirt. It felt like it stuck to my chest right away. To make sure it wasn't exposing my breasts, I tugged and pinched it. There wasn't much to see.

I yelled, slapping his palm firmly, "Stop it."

He came to an end. He apologized while holding up his wrist.

"Have I hurt you?" I asked, realizing instantly that I had screamed and smacked him so severely.

"It's okay," he murmured, taking his wrist off of him. "I was only having fun."

Something lodged in my throat. I told him, "I know, I'm not used to playing around." "I apologize for hitting you."

"I'll interpret it as a kiss." He smiled and put his wrist back.

I grabbed his hand and exclaimed, "I did hurt you."

Withdrawing, he said, "Don't bite it."

"Hand it over to me." I held up a hand motion. He did, and I applied pressure to ease his discomfort. He gave me a disapproving glance as I was working.

"I don't always skip things. Returning to the topic, he stated, "It's not easy to skip." "It must be planned ahead of time."

"Yes, how?" I inquired, holding onto his hand.

"Well, you must be aware of the phone number that will be used to inform them of your absence. You must be in charge of that voicemail. My residence is unoccupied during the day when the school calls. Furthermore, you must be aware of your destination. You can't just go to the parking lot, after all. I enjoy watching movies," he said. You must know the movie schedule, whether the professors will be suspicious, and what to do if you are discovered. Don't commit the crime if you can't serve the term.

I remarked, "You seem like a little mastermind."

"Yes, otherwise you're going to get caught," he stated gravely. "I do it once or twice a month, and I only skip the last two periods, not the full day. I sow the seed far in advance as well. I informed the teacher that I had an assignment due that day. They can then anticipate my absence.

I exclaimed, "Oh my god, you're a hoodlum." "Your innocence is deceiving."

He questioned, "Who said I looked innocent?"

How cute.

I inquired, "So, are you staying here for the summer?"

"Maybe longer, not sure." He stated.

"For how long?" I had great hopes when I asked.

"I'm not sure." He shrugged his shoulders and shifted uneasily. His face darkened.

I said, "Did something happen?"

He started to cry. "A little bit," he remarked.

"What took place?" I questioned while cradling his hand between mine.

He inhaled deeply. It's alright. My mother was arrested.

Unexpectedly, I let out a gasp.

"It's not the first time," he remarked, "It was kind of my fault this time because she was doing so well."

I questioned, "What do you mean it was your fault?"

He paused. "Well, at school, I kind of got into a fight."

I said, "You kind of got into a fight?"

Joel is this little child. Although he is very kind and intelligent, and my friend, other kids tease him when I'm not there," he remarked.

I questioned, "Why do they make fun of him?"

He remarked angrily, "Because they're bullies and stupid, and they only pick on the kids that don't fight back."

"I understand," I replied.

He added, "He's also autistic."

I understood and nodded.

He claimed, "This time they went too far; they shoved him to the ground in physical education and stole his underwear and shorts."

Squeezing his hand, I asked, "What did you do?"

"I was on the other side of the track, so I didn't see what happened," he stated. I spotted one of the kids running with Joel's shorts as I got to Joel and realized what had happened, so I chased after him.

Yes, I replied, my eyes wide.

"He bolted from the track in the direction of the classrooms. I tackled him after catching up to him halfway.

I asked, "Did you hit him?"

With tears, he replied, "I was so angry. How can they do that?" Not only was it unfair. I discovered that four of them restrained him while the other child removed his shorts.

"What transpired?" I queried.

"I punched him while seated on top of him after tackling him. He began to bleed—I mean, really bleed. As it happens, I broke his nose. I got blood all over my shirt and shorts; he was a mess. It appeared worse than it was. I only struck him once. He inhaled deeply. They made a huge fuss over it. They also called my mother and the cops. They dismissed her when she had to abandon her job to get to school. She claimed they were only seeking a reason to release her.

I asked, "Did you explain what the other kids did?"

Indeed, he replied. "All the other kids told the principal how the kids are really bullies and they always do this kind of stuff," I said, along with Joel. The principal had no interest in it. He said that I was to blame for striking the child.

That's normal, I said, explaining why bullies never quit. The school takes no action, and you will face consequences if you attempt to stop them.

Monkey stated, "That's exactly what happened."

However, how was your mother arrested? I enquired.

He said, "My mom had an issue with pain medication." After her vehicle accident, it turned into an addiction, and she was imprisoned for stealing. Drugs make you willing to do anything. She searched the driveway for bicycles that had been left outside and pawned them for fast cash to get high. After being discovered, she was imprisoned and released on a special probationary program. They test her at random to find out if she's still clean. The last time she failed, the sheriff showed up and handcuffed her right in front of me. It was awful. My mother is ill but otherwise fine. This is more than just a substance.

"Now, where's your mom?" "She will be incarcerated for three months. He stated. I answered, glancing at him, "I see." "You realize that this isn't in any way your fault, right?"

"If I hadn't struck the boy," he began.

"No, that's not how it works," I cut in. I apologize, but your mother is dealing with issues unrelated to you. It is a disease, as you mentioned. You do realize that you didn't cause her illness?

"No," he acknowledged.

"I believe that in order to assist your mother, you must put her needs ahead of your own. I smiled and said, "Monkey, it's not about you.

He explained, "It's just that she was doing so good."

I assured him, "Yes, and when she goes out and you're there to support her, I'm sure she'll do better."

"Anyway," he murmured. I'll be residing with my aunt till my mother is discharged. We will hunt for a new place to stay because we lost our flat.

"It would be wonderful if you could move in with your aunt. I'm visible to you every day.

"Why is that so amazing?" He smiled and said.

Are you trying to act aloof or distant? I informed him, shoving him with my shoulder, "Because you suck at it."

"My aunt suggested that as a possibility," he remarked. She's terrified about her mother. She sobs every night when she believes I'm not listening to her.

In response, I was at a loss for words.

I said, "So, what's your favorite subject?"

"You," he whispered, his gaze piercing. The tingles in my stomach got stronger. Butterflies.

"No, you fool. In school," I murmured, experiencing my first-ever blush. Could he notice that this light made me blush? I grabbed my hair's ends.

He gazed at the water while thinking for a short while. He declared, "I like world religions."

Global faiths? You don't have my trust. You don't go college, I remarked.

"It's not available at my school," he remarked. "I read it by myself. I also saw every video and listened to the library's recorded courses.

"What?" I asked, glancing at him oddly. I remained unconvinced.

Indeed, he replied, "I also take anthropology."

Anthropology, I questioned. "You are insane." This boy was peculiar. He acts like a youngster one minute, skipping and disparaging school. The other is more like a scholar. I can again feel comfortable about him.

What kind of literature do you enjoy? With particular attention, I turned to face him and inquired.

He added, "You know about how we grow and develop, about how we evolve emotionally."

"What?" I questioned. My hand began to sweat. He seemed to be my soul mate.

"You mean like how we become adults and learn new things?" or how our culture develops?" I asked.

He gave me a foolish little smile.

"I've got a theory," he declared. "More of an idea about our sideways reincarnation as a means of evolution."

I perked up and said, "More, more."

Thus, reincarnation is a belief held by several societies. After dying, you reincarnate into a different body. This indicates that the concept of the soul already exists. The soul can exist successively in multiple bodies. The issue is that you must pass away before you can reincarnate and take on a new body," he stated.

"I comply," I murmured. He was fully immersed in it. He researched this material.

Gazing downward into the shadows, Belial thought of how wonderful it would be to have a woman truly mean it when she declared her love for him and how he wanted to make everything right for Destiny. Swinging his body over the balcony railing, he fell about forty feet and landed like a cat, experiencing a brief, nebulous tremor of pain before it disappeared. He shot one more look at Destiny's window before turning and sprinting towards his car, which was parked on the side road near Blade House.

Section 4.

I was unable to unwind or fall back asleep after that dream. Rolling over, I checked the time on my alarm clock and was shocked to see that it was only midnight. At this point, I couldn't get up and start exploring the house, could I? Instead, I read a book that Marietta had lent me, and after a while, I was finally tired enough to fall asleep. I woke up at 6:15 a.m. and realized there was no way I could sleep again. I dressed in my old trousers and a cozy fleece top, pulled my hair back into a ponytail, and went downstairs.

Josh likes to get up early and go to bed late, so I wasn't surprised when he sat at our kitchen table solving the crossword from yesterday's newspaper. Josh can get by on around four hours of sleep every night. Ask not how!

"Good morning," I muttered as I sat across from him.

"Des, what did he do to you, hello?" Josh's eyes shone a gentle purple-blue light.

"Nothing is important anymore,"

"Perhaps a coffee would be nice for you?" Gently, he inquired.

It would be lovely to have hot chocolate with two sugars.

Josh sprung to his feet and moved with a predatory ease that fit him well. He continued to look at me while he mixed and poured my drink. Was there a possibility that he thought I might cut my wrists while he wasn't looking? When he returned, he put the hot chocolate mug in front of me and left it there briefly. He then repositioned himself to sit next to me around the table.

"Guys don't gossip either, and we listen really well too." He made a gentle proposition.

"I know that sometimes guys can be bigger bitches than girls, but are you okay with me telling you why I'm such a goose, Destiny?"

"I'm fine; just let Uncle Josh know," he said, smiling at me that I could not reciprocate.

"I was convinced that he was my soul mate, and I felt so right and loved in his arms. I just thought it was my chance to fall in love." Parallel streams of tears ran down my cheeks.

"You don't need Belial Di Aberlie, the stupid Yank; people here love you," Josh groaned as he hugged me and affectionately stroked my back. I raised my head and gazed into his eyes, not knowing if I had misunderstood him at that moment or if he had truly said, "I love you, Destiny." Give it a minute, Destiny! I placed my order. Don't make assumptions; Josh most likely wants to be your friend. I scolded myself.

"It must be love, I am crazy about you," Josh murmured once more, blushing profusely, but he didn't avert his gaze or do anything other than maintain his focus on me.

"Oh, Josh, I have no idea what to say." I muttered.

Josh made the kitchen seem like the most romantic location in the world, but for some reason, I never thought of it as a place to announce your unwavering love for someone. He kissed me properly after taking my hand and letting his lips glide over mine slowly, as though he was just giving me a taste. I tried to return the favor by accepting his offer and thought this kiss was very beautiful.

I was perplexed as I had always believed that I would discover my soul mate's identity the instant we shared a kiss. However, Josh and Belial experienced something far different from a typical kiss. God, oh God! What if I was one of those freaks who had two soul mates from birth? My mother would be here if only I could ask her for guidance.

"What are you considering?" Josh huskily mumbled.

"I'm perplexed...I'm not so sure now that I thought Belial was my soul mate. I acknowledged.

"I long to be your soul mate."

Although Josh had a reputation for being promiscuous, I knew he was also kind, and I wanted him to be too. And for as long as we lived together, I knew he would love me the way I needed to be loved. After expressing my wish for him to be as quick-witted as I was, he demonstrated his ability to think quickly enough.

However, how were you able to identify your soul mate? Do you believe a witch could be able to inform us? He asked, lightly touching my cheek.

I closed my eyes at his touch and said, "Maybe and there is that Witch shop up by the Erdington by the library - maybe we could try there."

I sensed his thoughts: could it be that he wasn't my soul mate? The problem was, I wasn't sure whether I could simply give up on the idea of soul mates, which my parents had instilled in me from a young age. Josh kissed me once more, seeking comfort from me and offering his wonderful comfort in return to ensure his feelings were not hurt.

Alec McKenzie, a twenty-six-year-old Witch Craft & Spells store employee, looked up as the bell on the door tinkled. Two vampires entered the room as he was waiting for Felicia, his coworker and lover, to return from her lunch break.

They looked so out of place here that Alec knew he would have recognized they weren't witches even if he hadn't sensed their vampire feelings.

"Is there anything I can do to help?" The male vampire gave him a short peek up as he inquired.

Seeing how they were merely staring at him, Alec was getting impatient. He sighed, went from the till area, and asked his query again, using the old language in case they were only speaking it.

"May I be of any assistance to you? Nadir contra fermatas de bocce?

"Hopefully so; we just need a basic spell." The man said, appearing irritated that Alec was speaking to him outdatedly.

And what kind of easy spell is that? I could name a few off the top of my head because so many are around these days. Was there a specific one you sought, or was it just a spell? Alec shot back with sarcasm.

"I need the spell, and I was wondering if there was a spell that could identify your soul mate based on the Soul Mate Principle." This time, the girl said nothing.

"I can't say I've ever heard of a spell to find your soul mate, but give me a moment, and I'll just check." Alec pivoted and passed through the intricately beaded curtain dividing the store from Sybille Grange, his employer and the proprietor, and her changing quarters at the rear. "Sybille? According to the principal, do spells exist to find a soul mate? A few vampires I know are asking for one. With grace, he questioned the older witch.

"Dead people? I'll see. Sybille went to the curtain and looked through the tinkling, wind-tossed beads. "I won't sell such a spell in this shop; it may exist on the black market, but it doesn't exist legally. Alec, if you'd like, I can take over. Locate Felicia; I believe she is upstairs in the apartment. Sybille gave her little trainee gentle instructions.

With gratitude, Alec hurried out, leaving Sybille to handle the vampire situation.

Sybille Grange fixed her well-groomed brown hair and entered the store, shocked to see how much the young man resembled her former partner, Belial Di

Aberlie. She knew Belial wouldn't know she was in England because she had traveled there from America, even if she hadn't seen him in decades. As the vampire dictator, he had made a great name for himself; as far as she knew, he was still single.

Could I help you in any way? I'm Sybille Grange, the chief witch and manager of this establishment. "You were looking for a spell to define a soul mate?" inquired my apprentice Alec. To the vampires, she said.

The attractive female vampire said, "It's me. I thought I had found my Soul mate, but now I am unsure because I've met someone else, and he strikes the same feeling, and I'm just looking for answers."

"Child, there isn't such a spell. I apologize, but is there any way I could sense your aura since that can be a very useful hint on its own? Sybille made a gentle proposition.

The girl trailed behind her to the rear chambers, where Sybille instructed her to have a seat while she obtained a pre-mixed aura disclosure spell from a storage area.

"Child, I feel like you already know how special a soul mate is. What was your name?" The spell was placed on the table in front of Sybille.

The girl answered, "Destiny Pane."

"Destiny Pane, I can't quite place why, but your name seems so familiar to me. Maybe I know your parents?"

The girl sighed regretfully, "Maybe you did, they died almost six years ago."

"Oh, child, I apologize," she said, gently patting her hands.

"I'm grateful,"

"A beautiful girl like you must have a million things to do this beautiful December morning. Let's get on with this aura reading." Sybille observed as the oily-feeling orange liquid turned into fine dust as she poured some of it into her palms. "Destiny, close your eyes. I can read your aura." After softly blowing the dust and observing it settle over the girl's shoulders, the girl's aura emerged, rising like a thin wisp of smoke.

"You have a wonderful future ahead of you, Destiny, with a man whose love will be very true when he finally accepts and forgets the past to trust in others. You are a very gentle girl." I see you will be quite happy shortly and have at least three lovely children, but oh my goodness, I also see danger and even a threat to someone you love, similar to the pleasure/pain theory where you are meant to live a long life. Fearfully, the halo disappears, and I can no longer see.

Sybille was filled with sadness as she realized that the man Destiny would eventually marry was her lost love since she had caught a glimpse of him. Refusing to accept the money Destiny attempted to offer as payment for her services, she led the girl back to her friend while remaining depressed over that vision. Then, she watched Destiny and her male friend leave before returning to her rooms to think and get back to her casting.

Chapter 14 JANACLESE

I sat on the park bench next to Hassan, slurping on a blue raspberry Slurpee and taking in every inch of him—gentle eyes, deep-set and inquisitive; full lips that smiled even when he seemed lost in thought; soft black hair curling at the nape of his neck.

Hassan stared back at me. Up close, a smooth band of hair barely peeked through his skin's surface and lightly lined his upper lip. Had he started shaving yet?

"You look like Nneka," he said.

What'd he mean by that? I bent my neck and looked up at him without lifting my head. "Your cute five-year-old sister?"

Indeed. You seem so innocent and carefree but with attractive blue lips."

My insides melted despite the solid mass my stomach carried. If he only knew the stuff going on in me.

"I'm glad I joined Redemption. So how come I didn't see you at the beginning of summer?"

"I was on a cultural tour of Costa Rica with my school. Then my mom set up a three-day mission for some of us with the Tico children."

Hassan leaned forward. "What was that like?"

"The tour was cool. Definitely an eye opener."

"No, tell me about your experience serving as a missionary in a foreign nation."

I got back up. "Ah, Hassan. I was enamored by it. Giving yourself to so many in need is a wonderful experience.

"Hmm ..." With a laugh, Hassan reclined on the bench.

"How about this one?"Cyndray called from the other side of the grass while examining a white wildflower. For some strange reason, she was continually inquiring about the scientific names of plants.

I exclaimed, "Lonicera," as I inhaled the sweet scent of honeysuckle lingering in the air.

"Are you familiar with plants?" Hassan got up and stretched for my hand.

"A few." I acted as though I didn't see his gesture. "Gardening is my mom's hobby.

She's around me a lot. Too much these days.

The honeysuckle, creeping along a hedge, was where we eased over to in Cyndray. "In the manner of this." I plucked the blossom off the bush, removed the stem, and sampled the delicious nectar. "Hmm, give it a shot."

"I'll pass, but you're really adorable." Again, Hassan stretched for my hand.

"With lips the color of blue? You're sinking quickly, boy. Cyndray grinned.

I let go of the flower and stood behind Cyndray, putting her between Hassan and myself.

At the rear of the park is a garden maze. Would any of you like to give it a try? My sisters find it to be really enjoyable. Hassan gestured to a wooden bridge connected to an entryway resembling a castle.

Cyndray looked at her timepiece. "It could take too long. We must return home quickly. Her eyebrows went up. "Before dusk."

Hassan's mouth twisted upward. "Oh, so you've heard about the local gangsters that operate after dark?"

I pursed my lips and turned to leave. They could at least make jokes about that stuff together.

"Hi, Shawty. Where are you going? Hassan called me.

"To the vehicle. I must return Cyndray home.

Hassan walked twice as fast as I was. "Oh, your signal light is flashing too quickly. Let me remind you of that."

There is a threat to the bulb. If you purchase a new one, I will swap it out.

"Gratitude." He kept the door open for me as I grinned and leaped into the driver's seat. "You really like to fix things, are you not?"

Cyndray wrenched open her door and climbed into the back seat as Hassan approached the side of his vehicle. She mumbled, "He needs to fix his raggedy truck."

Why was she attempting to complicate things for me? I mouthed, "Be nice," as I cast a quick peek at her in the rearview mirror.

Hassan gave a nod. "You're correct."

Was he speaking to me or Cyndray? I turned on the engine by pressing the power button. "So what will you do when you grow up if you're good at fixing things? A builder or an engineer? And please, don't say architect like my father did.

"None of the things mentioned above. I'm done with schooling. Eleventh grade is sufficient.

Cyndray gave a throat clearing. Another "I told you so" pricked my neck.

Hassan looked at me as I held the driving wheel with both hands. Your father is a building designer, while your mother is a gardener. Anything well-known?

Not really, though. There are a few buildings in the downtown area and our family's home. I took a swallow. Please, God, keep my parent's divorce from coming up.

"How about you?" Hassan squinted his eyes. "He kind of designed your house and buildings halfway through?"

I quickly looked in the rearview mirror and hoped Cyndray would change the topic. Miracle and I could tell when to give each other that cue. I threw up. Since the pool party, I haven't spent much time with Miracle. There were days when I felt unable to do anything without her.

"My family doesn't really live in the same house," Gripping the wheel, I did.

"Divorced?"

Divided.In the short term. I nibbled on my lip.

"It is not Mrs. Mitchell's garden." Cyndray's voice was filled with annoyance. She works in her own

Women's Wellness Center's garden. She spent years practicing law, putting criminals behind bars, before focusing on women's issues and providing free services to those in need.

"Did my mother give her resume to you last Tuesday evening?" My face reddened. When did she start hanging out with my mom so much?

"It was a great Tuesday night. Correct, Cyndray? For a brief while, Hassan looked at her as though they had a special relationship. I pursed my lips. What was the purpose of that?

Night fell smooth and gentle as we drove. The velvety dark sky was sprinkled with sparkles. On Hassan's street, I turned.

"Go by my residence. Let me show you something, please.

I carried on walking down the street.

"Park the car there and turn here." Hassan gestured to an empty lot.

There, in the backseat, Cyndray growled. Hassan, I knew you were a little strange. But why do you now act like a complete moron? We're returning home.

"Cyndray." You are aware that I won't be doing something foolish. Hassan spoke in a level tone. "You are familiar with me."

Did she?

Cyndray got out of the automobile, and I went with him.

"You discussed your mother's Center for Women in Need and your distant mission trip. All I wanted was for you to see the need in our town.

"Hassan, the light is out." We have nothing to see. Cyndray shook her head.

Just have a look. Take a moment to observe closely. Hassan put us to the test.

In the gloom, I focused. Then I noticed— shotgun homes dating back to the 1800s. My dad had architectural photos of these small-framed houses hanging on the wall of his workplace as a nod to his culture. Lights flickered in windows with no shades or drapes to protect their privacy. Kids wandered around without shoes or clothes, their bottoms tattered.

Cyndray took a circular route. What if some individuals prefer candlelight? They may find it romantic.

"Are you blind to the fact that they don't have electricity?" We have the doors open to let in the summer breeze because the interior is stuffy and heated. Some have removed the curtains to avoid a fire hazard since they cannot afford battery-operated flashlights. That dude over there, do you see him?

"Yes, I do see someone bending over." Cyndray froze where she was. "No, two individuals bending." A head lifted. "Are there any others?"

Many families in this part of town are without a place to live. They'll be alright through the summer until the next shift in weather.

My eyes suddenly broke into a spontaneous stream of tears. Unable to respond, I stared up into Hassan's questioning eyes. Was he criticizing me for not knowing better? Despite having so much to do at home, just across town from my lovely suburban life, we had worked so hard overseas.

I was unable to communicate the answer, so Hassan looked through Cyndray. "Did I make a mistake?"

"About Janaclese, huh."Cyndray tapped me on the shoulder. Hassan is quite sensitive. This is beyond her. It wasn't right of you to bring her here.

Cyndray was correct. I felt weak and powerless when I heard her declare that I couldn't handle what I'd seen. I dashed to my car to avoid taking on the responsibility of knowing.

I had my cheek pressed against my Prius' roof when Hassan arrived. He put his hands on my trembling shoulders and made me turn to face him.

"Hi there, you." He gave a headshake. "Shakoty, it's not your fault."

However, I— My effort at a cohesive sentence was cut off by sobs.

"Hush... " Hassan pulled his body closer to mine, putting his index finger to my lips. "Your living situation is unrelated to theirs. Are you aware of that?

He wiped the moisture from my cheeks while maintaining eye contact with me. My spine tingled as a different emotion was awakened by his delicate touch. He leaned forward, his face meeting yours, cheek to cheek. Every inch of my body tingled—my heart was beating quickly, my stomach was full of butterflies, and my lashes brushed against his.

I pursed my lips and closed my eyes. Holding out for...

"Way too much PDA, that." Cyndray's voice commandeered the scene.

Just as she was pushing Hassan away, I opened my eyes. She disliked showing affection in public.

"Seeing all of this makes me feel really bad," Cyndray remarked. But time has slipped from our grasp. We had to leave immediately and go home.

Twelve

"I cherish you." His voice was raspy from the anguish he was suppressing. He held his breath as he gazed into her face.

Would she forgive him for the hurt he had given her? After all this time, will she still love him?

She remained silent. She shook her head, grinning. It's too late, you say. She approached a tall man wearing a tan uniform and extended her hand.

She was gone by the time he realized it too late.

In his slumber, Mark murmured, "Vickie, don't go." "No."

Vickie called her name to him as she looked up from her book. Though she couldn't hear it in his speech, she could see the serenity on Mark's face. Where was she meant to have gone, she wondered. His eyes opened, and she saw him look around the room for her. His anxious eyes landed on her, and he let out a relieved breath.

"You remain here."

She felt warmer from the simple words than the flames directly before her. "Where should I have gone?" she inquired, nodding toward the half-drawn curtain. "It's freezing outside and snowing again."

"You departed." She put her book down after hearing his two-word response.

"I left because you allowed me to," She was becoming skilled at expressing her feelings to him. She was aware that there was more she could have said. However, it was all merely a dream; nothing was genuine.

"Vicki, I'm speaking of a dream. Nothing more. His speech had a gravelly tone that heightened the dramatic impression.

Vickie held herself back from continuing. She recalled the time he fractured his arm and was unable to play ball. Even though he had raged at her then, his mother had pulled her away. She clarified that he reacted aggressively because he disliked feeling unimportant or unwelcome. He resembled a wounded bear that needed to frighten everyone away in order to get healed.

She said, "Maybe you ought to be talking." "You know, I recall there were moments when you were eager to speak with me."

Mark cast a half-lidded glance at her. "Changes occurred."

She remarked, "Not as much as you think." Did you know that a law in Jasper Hill says you have to salute everyone you meet when riding a camel through the town? Or that on Mondays, you can take a soak in the Avery Fountain?

"Who would be insane enough to take a bath in front of everyone in the town square?"

"I'm not sure, but the law must have a purpose. I've read that Jasper enjoyed swimming every two to four weeks.

Mark grinned and remarked, "Imagine the stench that probably followed him."

"This is something I like."

Vickie wished there wasn't much more to be said after hearing those three words. But glancing at Mark, she realized that all those more serious talks would have to wait.

"You don't feel well at all, do you?" She rose from her floor-cushioned spot.

"Nope, my throat aches."

Vickie checked the medication cupboards to see if there was anything for a sore throat and cold. She told a closed-eyed Mark, "I'll be back," and walked off to see if she could get any medicine.

Thirteen

Vickie awoke two mornings later to music emanating from the tiny radio Mark had discovered in his suitcase. With the TV remote missing, it was their only connection to the outside world. She remained under her covers, warm and cozy, and lay there enjoying a song about popping happy pills. After the song concluded, a brief weather report aired. There was supposed to be a worse storm than the previous one.

"Goddammit!" She had to cover her mouth to keep him from hearing her chuckle as the expletives were whispered in her ear. "I assume you're awake?" It seemed as though he was feeling better.

Yesterday morning, she had become weary of attempting to converse with him. Since his cold had worsened, all she had heard him say were moans and single words. He had been grumpy and growly, much like a bear.

Vickie looked up into the man's face. The bear can say more than "yes" and "nope." He had been a terrible patient and roommate. And she would inform him about it.

With her hair ruffled and her eyes sparkling with amusement, Mark turned to face the woman lying on the ground. "Ha, ha," uttered he. "I guess that means I've been an animal for the past couple of days." He had been, he knew. He had felt terrible. His head had pounded, and his throat ached. He didn't want Vickie to see him that way, so he wished he had been elsewhere.

For the past few days, he had been thinking about a dream. She had moved on without him since he had arrived too late. He wasn't sure what his consciousness was trying to teach him or what he wanted to take away from the dream. Did he want to be with her, or did he fear that she would stop loving him if he didn't make the right decision quickly? Despite two days of reflection, his conflicted feelings persisted.

"Yes, you have," she said with a smile. "So, you're feeling better?" Thankfully, she couldn't stand the stillness or any more one-word responses.

"Today, I feel so much better. I may head outside to take a shower before the storm arrives. You never know when our hot water supply will run out due to an outage of electricity. He got to his feet and left the room.

As Vickie watched the man in the boxers walk away, she was reminded of the morning she had discovered him strapped to the bed. The wave of shame washed over her even now. In reality, she had touched his naked chest and straddled him. The fantasy ended with a kiss and lasted only for a few minutes. That kind of thought about him filled her heart with optimism.

♥♥♥

Standing in the mist, Mark prayed the impending storm wouldn't be as severe as forecast. He might need all the power he possessed today, so he was relieved to feel better.

When Vickie discovered the suitcase his brother had sent, he was overjoyed. He was eager to take off the princess sweatpants. After bringing the package inside, he examined the ribbons still fastened to the poles. He had dismissed the recollection they evoked.

After placing the suitcase on the bed, he took off his clothing. On the bottom, he had discovered a box with a note inside.

"On the off chance," his sibling had written. The Trojan box had been pushed back to the bottom by Mark. He hadn't been inclined to utilize them.

It was two days before that. He considered pulling out the package and presenting it to Vickie now. She had complete control over them; she could even blow them up if she desired. He would be insane to waste them that way, a voice in the recesses of his mind warned him.

He turned off the faucet and patted himself dry. He needed to bring in a lot of wood to keep the cottage warm all day and all night, so he dressed in jeans and a long-sleeved shirt.

Vickie was fast asleep when he came back into the living room. When he abruptly stopped walking, he saw that her legs were uncovered and that the covers were just partially pulled off. She had the best legs he'd seen in a long time, no question about it. He shook his head, attempting to banish those ideas from his consciousness.

After putting on the orange jacket and boots, he gathered some firewood.

♥♥♥

Chapter 9: Home, Drunken

With a fluff of her eyes, Trix opened them. Her eyes partially opened, and she stared at the strange wall, trying to recall what had happened the night before, where she was, and how she had gotten there. It was beyond midday when she noticed it from the light streaming in through the window.

B*tch.

Using one hand to prop herself up, she rubbed her head with the other. "I ought not to have taken that final shot."

Her clothing was piled on the floor as she opened her eyes. "Fuck, ugh!"

The incident from last night reappeared all at once.

"I ought to be the first person to go! Trix clenched her skull, "Ow."

She was able to recall everything. The dancing, flirting, and the flow of beverages. Before they made out in the club's rear and had sex, she flirted with the attractive man with the Buttery Nipple at the bar. Right here.Trix winced at the idea.

B*tch.B*tch.B*tch.

"How in the hell?" Her headache ached.

Something felt wrong, something she didn't like in her throat. With her mouth sealed shut, she bolted toward the restroom. She stumbled when the covers wrapped around her feet. She was unable to arrive in time. She quickly realized that she had puked all over the floor.

She muttered to herself, "Fucking great," and used the back of her hand to wipe her mouth.

But the sickening sensation was back.

She lurched to her feet and dashed to the bathroom.

Her stomach ache turned from a churning queasiness to a dull ache the more she heaved. With her head hanging over the ceramic bowl, she let out a cough and spat. All she could think of was saliva and bile stuck in her hair.

She forced herself to get up and flush the toilet once her stomach finally settled. After using a tissue to wipe her mouth, she threw the tissue in the garbage and found a used condom inside.

For a split second, she felt grossed out, but then relief came over her. Well, they did wear one.

She picked up the condom and filled it with water using a lot of tissue. No escapes. A sigh of relief left her.

With her body weak, Trix staggered back into the bedroom, straining her knees to sustain herself. With a lurch, she reached the side of the bed and collapsed, allowing her head to drop into her hands.

She thought about giving Olympia a call. She would be aware of how to handle this.

However, she made the decision not to. It seems that she left the bar later than she did. It wasn't right to bother her and force issues upon her. She would simply return to her slumber and ride this out.

Her tiredness and hangover were causing her eyelids to droop. It was difficult for her to keep them open. She had returned to sleep in a deep, dreamless sleep before realizing her eyelids were closed.

She awoke again to find everything completely dark.

She put on her clothes from last night and hurriedly left the room. That was how she liked it. Having a one-night stand with a stranger was better than having a committed relationship. She felt more than a little relieved.

As she left the inn, she called for a cab that was approaching. She didn't realize she was this far downtown. The trip back to her place was going to be quite the one.

Amid the several folders accumulated on her desk, TRIX GROWLED OVER ONE. With her head resting in her hands, she reclined in her chair and sighed.

Are you still suffering from a severe hangover, Trixie? Olympia had a playful smile as she stole a look into Trix's office.

Trix whispered between her hands, "Shut up, P."

Olympia chuckled and said, "I'll take that as a yes," before entering and closing the door. But what happened to you? You were out of reach for the entire day and never returned from the club's restroom!

"I'm doing great! After a difficult day, I only wanted to go to bed. Trix groaned.

"What took place with you? I was prepared to make a police report. Olympia became serious in her speech.

"What I did was incredibly stupid." Trix rubbed her forehead.

Olympia's expression twisted into a scowl as she comprehended Trix's meaning. "No!" she exclaimed.

She admitted, "I had a one-night stand with a stranger."

"What the fucking hell?" Olympia's jaw dropped agape. "I should have taken your inebriated ass home, I knew."

"I wasn't even too inebriated. Hence, I knew what I was doing. Trix sat back down, totally nonplussed. She waited, and their stillness lengthened. It was foolish. It's unbelievable that I did it.

It's alright. Likely, you won't see that guy again. Olympia dismissively waved her hand.

"What happens if I see him?"

When was the last time you were able to recall faces? I'm unsure how often you've made a fool of yourself by introducing yourself to people you've already met at parties.

"What do you know? You're correct, Trix concurred. She squints her eyes slightly. "I can now enjoy the advantages of my dyslexia."

How was it back then? Olympia took a seat in one of the seats facing Trix's desk. "Getting intimate with an unfamiliar person."

Trix closed her eyes and encircled her arms about herself. It was intense. My body felt as though it had melted into him, trapping me. There wasn't enough space in my senses to be attentive to anything else but him.

Olympia's lips were pursed. Was he hot, then?

Trix grinned. "Yes, my dear," All across her face was flush.

Pauline walked in and hovered over Trix's desk, saying, "Conference room in five."

"Bitches, be warned, Thompson is having a rough day. Be careful."

Trix mumbled, "Oh great," and used all her power to push herself off her desk.

Olympia smirked as they walked into the conference room, saying, "I guess we'll have to continue this conversation a little later."

The engagement level of each department was discussed, along with the potential acquisition of their primary rival, the Wilton Patel company, in TODAY'S AGENDA. Join them if you can't defeat them. An infamous legal tactic to end shady business dealings.

With a worried smile, Trix nodded to the other department heads as she entered the meeting room.

The head of the administration and finance department, Ms. Colton, questioned, "Should we get started?"

The CEO, Mr. Thompson, took up half of the room and stood in the center of the long oak table. On either side of him were the remaining department heads. He scowled everyone.

"Financial losses have arisen with more expenses incurred, with reports suggesting increasing opposition by certain insurers." The room was filled with the monotonous voice of Mr. Thompson. The silence that fell was a testament to the tension in the room. It would have made even the sound of a needle landing on the floor seem louder.

Mr. Thompson scowled at the head of the Sales Department, Jason Walker, also known as Mr. Giga, who believed he was smarter than everyone else. He knew how the world should work and was always right, and everyone else was wrong.

The CEO went on, "People, things are not good." "Miss Moreno." Everyone looked at Trix.

The company raised funds because of Trix's marketing methods and first-hand experience, making it Perth's top financial services company.

Yes, Mr. Thompson, please. Trix lost consciousness. She straightened her seat right away.

"Work in tandem with the Sales Division. The sales and marketing team must collaborate and function as a unit.

The chief of customer services, Mr. Nguyen, remarked, "Traits they clearly lack."

"I'm going to implement a new program now. Trix said, "The marketing team often grips about the salespeople 'doing their own thing' and not adhering to the overall strategy.

"Please forgive me." Taken aback by the slur, Trix looked at him in shock. Are you referring to indolent theorists?

"The board has been keeping an eye on your work. It has been difficult for your department to present positive numbers. Additionally, Moreno, there's that 32% drop in revenue. Jason gave Trix a look as he fixed him with his gaze.

"What do you mean by that?" Trix tightened her jaw. Jason made a valid argument, but Trix would sooner die than acknowledge it.

"Moreno, please keep your matters out of the business. Jason glared at her, saying, "You're taking down all of us."

The CEO said, "Get your asses out and take your fight outside."

I apologize, Mr. Thompson. Jason took a seat again.

Trix's expression twisted into a furious one as she viewed the slide displaying her department's dismal output. How embarrassing as well as irritating!

Trix averted his gaze but met Jason's eyes. A "I won" grin sprang on his face.

God, he is the devil's offspring. I detest him!

She required a change of scenery.

Using her laptop, Trix launched a browser and perused her social media accounts. Her gaze was constantly fixed on her laptop, avoiding the presentation on the wall directly before her.

Her newsfeed flashed the latest Ford Mustang model. Her heart skipped a beat in anticipation of an automobile. Trix had excellent managerial abilities and was good with people, money, and numbers. However, Trix was a master car mechanic in his heart. She was just so damned good at it. Back in the Philippines, her father had a car repair business. She grew up surrounded by cars, so it came easy to her.

She enjoyed troubleshooting automotive issues and could immediately tell what was wrong with a car based only on its feel, sight, smell, and sound. She was capable of problem-solving, assessment, and even car reassembling.

Trix continued to read through her feed until she came across an advertisement for a fully functional, independently owned auto repair shop that was up for sale.

Mr. Thompson and the others got to their feet. She stood in line to usher everyone out of the conference room. She closed her laptop, saved the advertisement, and left the room with the ridiculous-looking board members.

9 781835 733530